HYPERTHYROIDISM JUICING RECIPES BOOK

Harness the Healing Power of Fruits and Vegetables: Nutritious Juices for a Healthy Thyroid

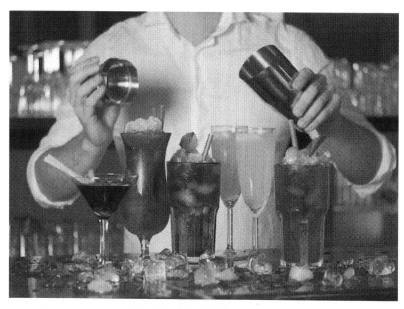

Dr Khady White

COPYRIGHT

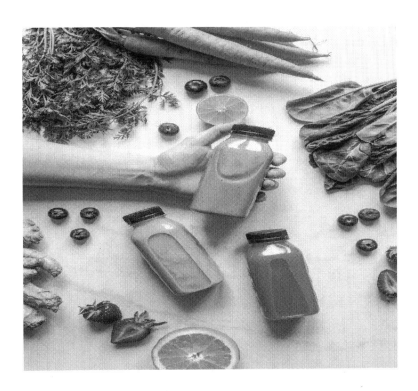

TABLE OF CONTENT

INTRODUCTION

Hyperthyroidism is a condition that occurs when the thyroid gland produces an excessive amount of thyroid hormones. This can lead to a variety of symptoms, including weight loss, rapid heartbeat, anxiety, and increased sensitivity to heat. While medical intervention is crucial for managing hyperthyroidism, adopting a healthy lifestyle and incorporating nutritious foods into your diet can also play a supportive role in managing the condition. One such approach gaining popularity is juicing.

Juicing involves extracting the liquid from fruits, vegetables, and herbs to create a concentrated beverage packed with essential vitamins, minerals, and antioxidants. These nutrients can provide numerous benefits for individuals with hyperthyroidism by supporting overall health and promoting a balanced thyroid function.

4

In this article, we will explore the potential benefits of juicing for hyperthyroidism and how it can be incorporated into a well-rounded approach to managing the condition. We will discuss specific fruits, vegetables, and herbs that may be particularly beneficial, as well as some important considerations to keep in mind when juicing for hyperthyroidism. It is important to note that while juicing can be a valuable addition to a healthy lifestyle, it is not a substitute for medical treatment or professional advice. Consulting with a healthcare professional is crucial for developing an individualized plan that suits your specific needs.

So, if you're interested in learning how juicing can support your overall health and help manage hyperthyroidism, read on to discover the potential benefits and delicious recipes that can assist you on your journey to optimal well-being!

CHAPTER ONE

Overview of Hyperthyroidism

Hyperthyroidism is an endocrine disorder that affects the thyroid gland, located in the throat area, which regulates the metabolic rate of the body. It is the result of overproduction of thyroid hormones; usually triiodothyronine (T3) and thyroxine (T4) from the thyroid gland. Hyperthyroidism is a condition that is becoming more common. Although it is evermore prevalent, many people are still unaware of its symptoms and treatments.

The main symptom of hyperthyroidism is a hypermetabolic state which is a result of an overproduction of thyroid hormones. Symptoms may include increased heart rate, weight loss, nervousness, fatigue, irritability, and anxiety. Other weight and menstrual changes, vision problems, and goiter (enlargement of the thyroid glands) can also be associated with hyperthyroidism.

The cause of hyperthyroidism tends to vary and is typically divided into two categories: autoimmune and non-autoimmune etiologies. Graves Disease, an autoimmune disorder, is the most common cause of hyperthyroidism. Non-autoimmune hyperthyroidism can be attributed to a multinodular goiter or toxic adenoma, both of which are conditions that cause excessive production of hormones. Additionally, taking too much of replacement hormones, such as levothyroxine, can also cause hyperthyroidism.

Diagnosis of hyperthyroidism typically begins with a physical exam and a lab test to measure thyroid hormone levels in the blood (TSH, T3, T4). Other tests, such as an Imaging scan, may also be done to check for any structural abnormalities of the thyroid gland.

Hyperthyroidism is a treatable condition and the goal of treatment is to reduce the amount of thyroid hormone the body produces. Treatments usually involve taking anti-thyroid medications to reduce the level of thyroid hormones produced, radioactive iodine to reduce thyroid activity, and sometimes thyroid surgery to remove part or all of the thyroid gland. Beta-blockers may also be recommended to help reduce symptoms such as rapid heart rate. In addition to the aforementioned treatments, patients may need to adjust their diets to limit foods that contain iodine and may need to use nutritional supplements to account for any deficiencies created by the thyroid hormones.

Hyperthyroidism does not have to be a serious, life-altering illness. With the proper diagnosis and treatment, it can be managed efficiently, allowing those with the disorder to live a normal life. By educating yourself and communicating with your doctor, you can work together to ensure that you have the best treatment for your specific condition.

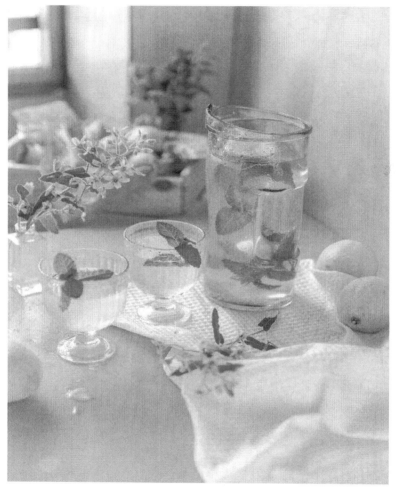

CHAPTER TWO

Causes of Hyperthyroidism

1. Graves' Disease: An autoimmune disorder where the body's immune system mistakenly attacks the thyroid gland, causing it to produce too much thyroid hormone

2. Toxic Multinodular Goiter: Usually benign nodules form in the thyroid which produces too many hormones.

3. Subacute Thyroiditis: Temporary inflammation of the thyroid gland that causes it to become overactive.

4. Excess Ingestion of Iodine: Too much iodine in the diet can cause the thyroid to become overactive and produce too much thyroid hormone.

5. Taking Too Much Thyroid Hormone: For individuals taking thyroid hormone replacement therapy, dosing errors can lead to hyperthyroidism.

6. Certain Medications: Certain medications such as amiodarone and interferon can cause the thyroid to become overactive.

7. Pituitary Hyperfunction: An enlargement of the pituitary gland in the brain can cause it to produce too much TSH which in turn causes the thyroid to become overactive.

8. Thyroid Adenomas: Benign tumors of the thyroid gland that can begin producing excess hormone.

9. Congenital Hyperthyroidism: A rare genetic disorder where an infant is born with an overactive thyroid.

10. Radioactive Iodine Treatment: Too much radioactive iodine used to treat

hyperthyroidism can cause the gland to become too active.

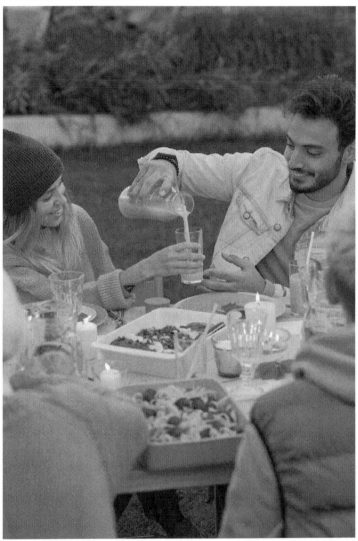

CHAPTER THREE

Symptoms of Hyperthyroidism

- Rapid heartbeat: Hyperthyroidism can cause an increased heart rate, leading to palpitations or a sensation of a racing heart.

- Weight loss: Despite having a normal or increased appetite, individuals with hyperthyroidism often experience unexplained weight loss.

- Increased appetite: Some people with hyperthyroidism may feel constantly hungry and have an increased desire for food.

- Nervousness and irritability: Excessive thyroid hormone levels can affect the nervous system, leading to feelings of restlessness, anxiety, and irritability.

- Fatigue and weakness: Despite experiencing an increased metabolism, individuals with hyperthyroidism often feel fatigued and weak.

- Difficulty sleeping: Insomnia or trouble falling asleep can be a symptom of hyperthyroidism, as the condition can interfere with normal sleep patterns.

- Heat intolerance: People with hyperthyroidism may find themselves more sensitive to heat, feeling excessively warm even in normal temperatures.

- Excessive sweating: Sweating more than usual, particularly in the palms of the hands or on the forehead, can be a symptom of hyperthyroidism.

- Tremors and muscle weakness: Hyperthyroidism can lead to trembling hands, particularly noticeable during activities that require fine motor skills.

- Changes in menstrual cycle: Women with hyperthyroidism may experience irregular menstrual periods, lighter flow, or even a complete cessation of menstruation.

It's important to note that these symptoms can vary from person to person, and some individuals may not experience all of them. If you suspect you have hyperthyroidism or are experiencing any of these symptoms, it is necessary to consult with a healthcare professional for a proper diagnosis and treatment.

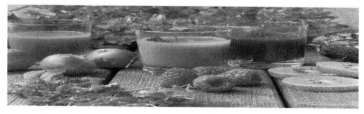

CHAPTER FOUR

Benefits of Juicing for the Management and Control of Hyperthyroidism

Juicing is a popular method of extracting nutrients from fruits and vegetables, and it can offer several benefits for overall health and well-being. When it comes to managing hyperthyroidism, a condition characterized by an overactive thyroid gland, juicing can provide some advantages as part of a comprehensive treatment plan. Here are the benefits of juicing and how it can support the management of hyperthyroidism:

- Increased nutrient intake: Juicing allows you to consume a concentrated amount of essential vitamins, minerals, and antioxidants found in fruits and vegetables. These nutrients can help support the overall health of your body, including your thyroid gland.

- Reduced inflammation: Many fruits and vegetables used in juicing, such as leafy greens, cucumbers, and berries, have anti-inflammatory properties. Inflammation can worsen the symptoms of hyperthyroidism, so including these ingredients in your juice can help reduce inflammation and promote healing.

- Support for immune function: Hyperthyroidism can weaken the immune system, making you more susceptible to infections and illnesses. Juicing nutrient-dense fruits and vegetables, especially those rich in vitamin C and antioxidants, they can strengthen your immune system and enhance your body's ability to fight off infections.

- Improved digestion: Hyperthyroidism can sometimes lead to digestive issues like diarrhea or increased bowel movements. Juicing can be beneficial for individuals with hyperthyroidism as it provides a concentrated dose of easily digestible nutrients, aiding in proper digestion and absorption of essential nutrients.

- Hydration and detoxification: Juicing can contribute to hydration, which is crucial for overall health and thyroid function. Proper hydration helps maintain the balance of hormones in the body and supports the elimination of toxins. Adding hydrating ingredients like cucumber or celery to your juice can assist in the detoxification process.

- Weight management: Hyperthyroidism can often result in unintended weight loss due to an increased metabolic rate. Juicing can provide a calorie-controlled option to help maintain a healthy weight by incorporating nutrient-dense ingredients into your diet without overloading on calories.

However, it's important to note that juicing should not replace a balanced diet or medical treatment for hyperthyroidism. It is always advisable to consult with your healthcare provider before making any significant dietary changes or incorporating juicing into your routine. They can provide personalized guidance and ensure it aligns with your condition and treatment plan.

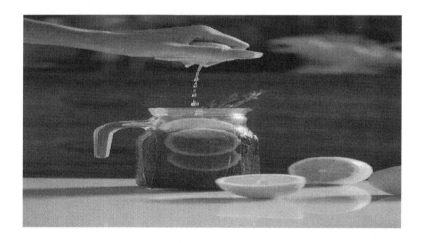

CHAPTER FIVE

Tips on Juicing for Hyperthyroidism

- Consult with a healthcare professional: Before making any significant changes to your diet, especially if you have a medical condition like hyperthyroidism, it's crucial to consult with a healthcare professional or a registered dietitian. They can provide personalized guidance based on your needs.

- Focus on cruciferous vegetables: Cruciferous vegetables such as kale, broccoli, cauliflower, and Brussels sprouts contain compounds that can support thyroid health. Include these vegetables in your juices as they are rich in nutrients and provide antioxidants.

- Use iodine-rich ingredients: Iodine is essential for thyroid function. Include iodine-rich ingredients in your juices, such as seaweed, dulse, and iodized salt, but be mindful of your overall iodine intake, as excessive amounts can be harmful.

- Include anti-inflammatory foods: Hyperthyroidism often involves inflammation in the body. Include ingredients with anti-inflammatory properties in your juices, such as turmeric, ginger, and berries, which can help reduce inflammation.

- Opt for low-sugar fruits: While fruits are generally nutritious, some can be higher in natural sugars. Choose low-sugar fruits like berries, green apples, and citrus fruits to avoid excessive sugar intake, which may affect blood sugar levels.

- Avoid goitrogenic foods: Goitrogens are substances that can interfere with thyroid function. Some examples include raw cruciferous vegetables, soy products, and certain nuts. Cooking these foods can help reduce their goitrogenic effects, but it's advisable to limit them in your juices.

- Include healthy fats: Healthy fats like avocado, coconut oil, and flaxseed oil can help support thyroid function and hormone balance. Add a small amount of these fats to your juices to enhance nutrient absorption.

- Consider juicing with herbs: Certain herbs like parsley, cilantro, and mint have potential benefits for thyroid health. Experiment with incorporating these herbs into your juices for added flavor and potential health benefits.

- Avoid excessive juicing: Juicing can be a healthy addition to your diet, but it's important to maintain a balanced approach. Juicing should not replace whole foods or a well-rounded diet. Consume juices as part of a varied and nutritious eating plan.

- Monitor your symptoms: Keep track of how your body responds to the juices. Monitor your energy levels, digestion, and any changes in symptoms related to your hyperthyroidism. If you notice any adverse effects or concerns, consult your healthcare professional for further guidance.

Remember, while juicing can be a beneficial way to incorporate nutrients into your diet, it's essential to maintain a well-rounded approach to nutrition and work in conjunction with healthcare professionals to manage your hyperthyroidism effectively.

CHAPTER SIX

JUICING RECIPES

- **Green Thyroid Tonic:**

Ingredients:

1 cucumber,

2 cups spinach,

1 green apple,

1/2 lemon (juiced)

Method:

Wash and juice all the ingredients together and enjoy.

- **Carrot and Beet Blend:**

Ingredients:

2 carrots,

1 small beet,

1-inch ginger root

Method:

Wash and then, juice all the ingredients together and drink it fresh.

- **Kale and Pineapple Delight:**

Ingredients:
2 cups kale,
1 cup pineapple,
1 cucumber
Method:
Wash and then, juice all the ingredients and
serve chilled.

- **Cooling Cucumber Lemonade:**

Ingredients:
2 cucumbers,
1 lemon (juiced), and a
handful of fresh mint leaves
Method:
Juice the cucumbers, then mix in the lemon
juice. Add mint leaves for extra freshness.

- **Berry Blast:**

Ingredients:
1 cup blueberries,
1 cup strawberries,
1 cup raspberries,
1 cup almond milk
Method:

Blend all the ingredients until smooth and enjoy.

- **Gingered Carrot Juice:**

Ingredients:

4 carrots,

1-inch ginger root,

1 apple

Method:

Juice all the ingredients and serve over ice.

- **Spinach and Celery Green Juice:**

Ingredients:

2 cups spinach,

3 celery stalks,

1 green apple,

1 lemon (juiced)

Method:

Juice all the ingredients together and serve chilled.

- **Apple and Cabbage Refresher:**

Ingredients:

2 green apples,

1/4 small green cabbage,
1 cucumber
Method:
Juice all the ingredients and enjoy.

- **Pineapple and Turmeric Elixir:**

Ingredients:
1 cup pineapple,
1-inch turmeric root,
1 orange (juiced)
Method:
Juice the pineapple and turmeric, then mix in the orange juice.

- **Carrot and Orange Medley:**

Ingredients:
4 carrots,
2 oranges (juiced),
1-inch ginger root
Method:
Juice the carrots and ginger, then mix in the orange juice.

- **Sweet Potato Surprise:**

Ingredients:

1 medium sweet potato,

2 carrots,

1 apple,

1-inch ginger root

Method:

Juice all the ingredients together and drink it fresh.

- **Cooling Cucumber Mint Juice:**

Ingredients:

2 cucumbers,

a handful of fresh mint leaves,

1 lime (juiced)

Method:

Juice the cucumbers, then mix in the mint leaves and lime juice.

- **Beet and Berry Blend:**

Ingredients:

1 small beet,

1 cup strawberries,

1 cup raspberries,

1 cup coconut water

Method:

Blend all the ingredients until smooth and enjoy.

- **Spinach and Pineapple Green Juice:**

Ingredients:

2 cups spinach,

1 cup pineapple,

1 cucumber,

1 lemon (juiced)

Method:

Juice all the ingredients and serve chilled.

- **Carrot and Parsley Cleanser:**

Ingredients:

4 carrots,

a handful of fresh parsley,

1 apple

Method:

Juice all the ingredients together and serve over ice.

- **Gingered Pear Juice:**

Ingredients:

2 pears, 1-inch ginger root,

1 lemon (juiced)

Method:

Juice the pears and ginger, then mix in the lemon juice.

- **Blueberry and Spinach Smoothie:**

Ingredients:

1 cup blueberries,

2 cups spinach,

1 banana,

1 cup almond milk

Method:

Blend all the ingredients until smooth and enjoy.

- **Radish and Cucumber Cooler:**

Ingredients:

4 radishes,

1 cucumber,

a handful of fresh cilantro,

1 lime (juiced)

Method:

Juice the radishes and cucumber, then mix in the cilantro and lime juice.

- **Beet and Carrot Elixir:**

Ingredients:

1 small beet,

2 carrots,

1 orange (juiced),

1-inch ginger root

Method:

Juice the beet and carrots, then mix in the orange juice and ginger.

- **Green Apple and Celery Juice:**

Ingredients:

2 green apples,

3 celery stalks,

1 cucumber,

1 lemon (juiced)

Method:

Juice all the ingredients together and serve chilled.

- **Orange and Ginger Zinger:**

Ingredients:

4 oranges (juiced),

1-inch ginger root

Method:

Juice the oranges, then mix in the ginger juice.

- **Mixed Berry Smoothie:**

Ingredients:

1 cup mixed berries (strawberries, blueberries, raspberries),

1 banana,

1 cup coconut water

Method:

Blend all the ingredients until smooth and enjoy.

- **Cooling Cucumber and Melon Refresher:**

Ingredients:

1 cucumber,

1 cup melon (watermelon or honeydew),

a handful of fresh mint leaves, 1 lime (juiced)

Method:

Juice the cucumber and melon, then mix in the mint leaves and lime juice.

- **Carrot and Spinach Elixir:**

Ingredients:

4 carrots,

2 cups spinach,

1 apple,

1 lemon (juiced)

Method:

Juice all the ingredients together and drink it fresh.

- **Pineapple and Ginger Zest:**

Ingredients:

2 cups pineapple,

1-inch ginger root,

1 orange (juiced)

Method:

Juice the pineapple and ginger, then mix in the orange juice.

- **Blueberry and Kale Green Juice:**

Ingredients:

1 cup blueberries,

2 cups kale,

1 cucumber,

1 lemon (juiced)

Method:

Juice all the ingredients and serve chilled.

- **Cucumber and Mint Lemonade:**

Ingredients:

2 cucumbers, a handful of fresh mint leaves,

2 lemons (juiced),

1 tablespoon honey (optional)

Method:

Juice the cucumbers and mint leaves, then mix in the lemon juice. Add honey to sweeten.

- **Carrot and Beet Boost:**

Ingredients:

2 carrots,

1 small beet,

1 orange (juiced),
1-inch ginger root
Method:
Juice the carrots and beet, then mix in the orange juice and ginger.

- **Green Goddess Juice:**
Ingredients:
2 cups spinach,
1 green apple,
1 cucumber,
1 lime (juiced)
Method:
Juice all the ingredients together and serve chilled.

- **Pineapple and Mint Refresher:**
Ingredients:
2 cups pineapple,
a handful of fresh mint leaves,
1 lime (juiced)
Method:
Juice the pineapple, then mix in the mint leaves and lime juice.

- **Carrot and Ginger Zinger:**

Ingredients:

4 carrots,

1-inch ginger root,

1 orange (juiced)

Method:

Juice the carrots and ginger, then mix in the orange juice.

- **Cooling Cucumber and Kiwi Juice:**

Ingredients:

2 cucumbers,

2 kiwis,

1 lemon (juiced)

Method:

Juice the cucumbers and kiwis, then mix in the lemon juice.

- **Green Energy Boost:**

Ingredients:

2 cups kale,

1 green apple,

1 cucumber,

1 lemon (juiced)

Method:

Juice all the ingredients together and serve chilled.

- **Beet and Orange Medley:**

Ingredients:

1 small beet,

2 oranges (juiced),

1-inch ginger root

Method:

Juice the beet and ginger, then mix in the orange juice.

- **Blueberry and Spinach Power Juice:**

Ingredients:

1 cup blueberries,

2 cups spinach,

1 green apple,

1 lemon (juiced)

Method:

Juice all the ingredients and serve chilled.

- **Carrot and Celery Cleanser:**

Ingredients:

4 carrots,

3 celery stalks,

1 apple,

1 lemon (juiced)

Method:

Juice all the ingredients together and serve over ice.

- **Pineapple and Turmeric Elixir:**

Ingredients:

2 cups pineapple,

1-inch turmeric root,

1 orange (juiced),

1 lemon (juiced)

Method:

Juice the pineapple and turmeric, then mix in the orange and lemon juice.

- **Green Power Smoothie:**

Ingredients:

2 cups spinach,

1 green apple,

1 banana,

1 cup almond milk,

1 tablespoon almond butter

Method:

Blend all the ingredients until smooth and enjoy.

- **Gingered Pear and Celery Juice:**

Ingredients:

2 pears,

3 celery stalks,

1-inch ginger root,

1 lemon (juiced)

Method:

Juice all the ingredients together and drink it fresh.

- **Cooling Cucumber and Lime Refresher:**

Ingredients:

2 cucumbers,

1 lime (juiced),

a handful of fresh mint leaves

Method:
Juice the cucumbers, then mix in the lime juice.
Add mint leaves for extra freshness.

- **Carrot and Orange Zest:**

Ingredients:
4 carrots,
2 oranges (juiced),
1-inch **ginger root**

Method:
Juice the carrots and ginger, then mix in the orange juice.

- **Berry Blast Smoothie:**

Ingredients:
1 cup mixed berries (strawberries, blueberries, raspberries),
1 banana,
1 cup coconut water,
1 tablespoon chia seeds

Method:
Blend all the ingredients until smooth and enjoy.

- **Kale and Green Apple Juice:**

Ingredients:

2 cups kale,

2 green apples,

1 cucumber,

1 lemon (juiced)

Method:

Juice all the ingredients and serve chilled.

- **Carrot and Parsley Green Elixir:**

Ingredients:

4 carrots, a handful of fresh parsley,

1 apple,

1 lemon (juiced)

Method:

Juice all the ingredients together and serve over ice.

- **Pineapple and Ginger Cooler:**

Ingredients:

2 cups pineapple,

1-inch ginger root,

1 orange (juiced)

Method:
Juice the pineapple and ginger, then mix in the orange juice.

- **Blueberry and Spinach Detox Juice:**

Ingredients:
1 cup blueberries,
2 cups spinach,
1 cucumber,
1 lemon (juiced),
1 tablespoon flaxseed
Method:
Juice all the ingredients and serve chilled.

- **Cooling Cucumber and Watermelon Refresher:**

Ingredients:
2 cucumbers,
1 cup watermelon,
a handful of fresh mint leaves,
1 lime (juiced)
Method:

Juice the cucumbers and watermelon, then mix in the mint leaves and lime juice.

- **Carrot and Beetroot Energizer:**

Ingredients:

2 carrots,

1 small beet,

1 orange (juiced),

1-inch ginger root

Method:

Juice the carrots and beet, then mix in the orange juice and ginger.

- **Green Immunity Booster:**

Ingredients:

2 cups spinach,

1 green apple,

1 cucumber,

1 lemon (juiced),

1 tablespoon honey (optional)

Method:

Juice all the ingredients together and serve chilled. Add honey to sweeten if desired.

- **Pineapple and Mint Green Juice:**

Ingredients:

2 cups pineapple,

a handful of fresh mint leaves,

1 lime (juiced)

Method:

Juice the pineapple, then mix in the mint leaves and lime juice.

- **Carrot and Ginger Energizing Juice:**

Ingredients:

4 carrots,

1-inch ginger root,

1 orange (juiced),

1 lemon (juiced)

Method:

Juice the carrots and ginger, then mix in the orange and lemon juice.

- **Cooling Cucumber and Kiwi Refresher:**

Ingredients:

2 cucumbers,

2 kiwis,

1 lemon (juiced), and

a handful of fresh basil leaves

Method:

Juice the cucumbers and kiwis, then mix in the lemon juice.

Add basil leaves for extra flavor.

- **Green Detox Smoothie:**

Ingredients:

2 cups kale,

1 green apple,

1 banana,

1 cup coconut water,

1 tablespoon spirulina powder

Method:

Blend all the ingredients until smooth and enjoy.

- **Beet and Orange Zinger:**

Ingredients:

1 small beet,

2 oranges (juiced),

1-inch ginger root

Method:
Juice the beet and ginger, then mix in the orange juice.

- **Blueberry and Spinach Hydrator:**

Ingredients:
1 cup blueberries,
2 cups spinach,
1 cucumber,
1 lemon (juiced),
1 cup coconut water

Method:
Juice all the ingredients and serve chilled.

- **Carrot and Celery Cleansing Juice:**

Ingredients:
4 carrots,
3 celery stalks,
1 apple,
1 lemon (juiced), and
a pinch of cayenne pepper (optional)

Method:

Juice all the ingredients together and serve over ice. Add a pinch of cayenne pepper for an extra kick if desired.

- **Pineapple and Turmeric Tonic:**

Ingredients:

2 cups pineapple,

1-inch turmeric root,

1 orange (juiced),

1 lemon (juiced),

a pinch of black pepper

Method:

Juice the pineapple and turmeric, then mix in the orange and lemon juice.

Add a pinch of black pepper to enhance turmeric's benefits.

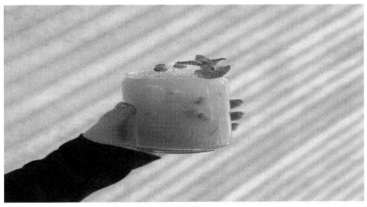

CONCLUSION

Juicing for Hyperthyroidism

In conclusion, juicing can be a beneficial addition to a comprehensive approach to managing hyperthyroidism. While it is not a cure or a standalone treatment, juicing can support overall health and provide essential nutrients that are beneficial for thyroid function. The key is to focus on juicing ingredients that are known to be beneficial for the thyroid gland and to consult with a healthcare professional before making any significant changes to your diet or treatment plan.

Hyperthyroidism is a complex condition that requires medical attention and personalized treatment. Juicing should be viewed as a complementary strategy to be used in conjunction with other conventional treatments and lifestyle modifications. It can offer a convenient and efficient way to increase the intake of nutrients that are important for thyroid health, such as iodine, selenium, and vitamins A, C, and E.

One of the main advantages of juicing is that it allows for the consumption of a variety of fruits, vegetables, and herbs in a concentrated form. These ingredients are rich in antioxidants and phytonutrients that have been shown to support the immune system and reduce inflammation, both of which are important for managing hyperthyroidism. For example, cruciferous vegetables like kale and broccoli contain compounds that can help regulate thyroid function and metabolism.

Additionally, juicing can provide a quick and easy way to incorporate thyroid-supportive herbs into your diet, such as ashwagandha, lemon balm, and bugleweed. These herbs have been traditionally used to support thyroid health and can be included in juicing recipes to harness their benefits.

However, it is crucial to note that juicing should not replace a balanced diet. Whole foods, including whole fruits and vegetables, contain valuable dietary fiber that is often lost during the juicing process. Fiber is important for digestive health and can help regulate blood sugar levels, which is especially important for individuals with hyperthyroidism.

It is essential to be mindful of the potential risks associated with juicing for hyperthyroidism. Certain foods and ingredients commonly used in juicing, such as goitrogenic vegetables like cabbage and kale, may interfere with thyroid hormone synthesis in some individuals. Therefore, it is important to consult with a healthcare professional who can provide personalized advice and guidance based on your specific condition.

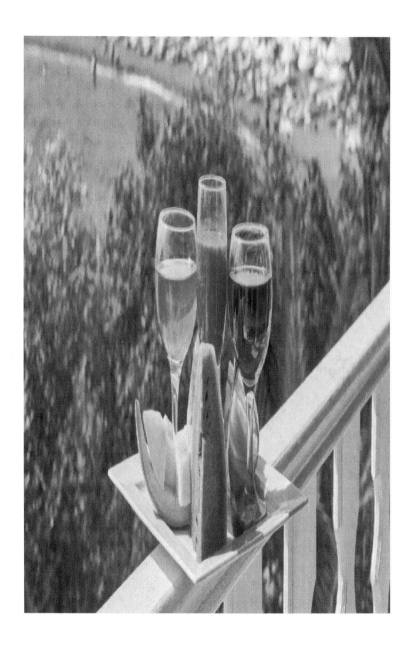

Made in the USA
Columbia, SC
19 June 2024

37278837R00028